# Vegetarian Anti-Inflammatory Recipes

*Protect Your Body with the Ultimate Collection of Veggie and Fast Meals*

Camila Allen

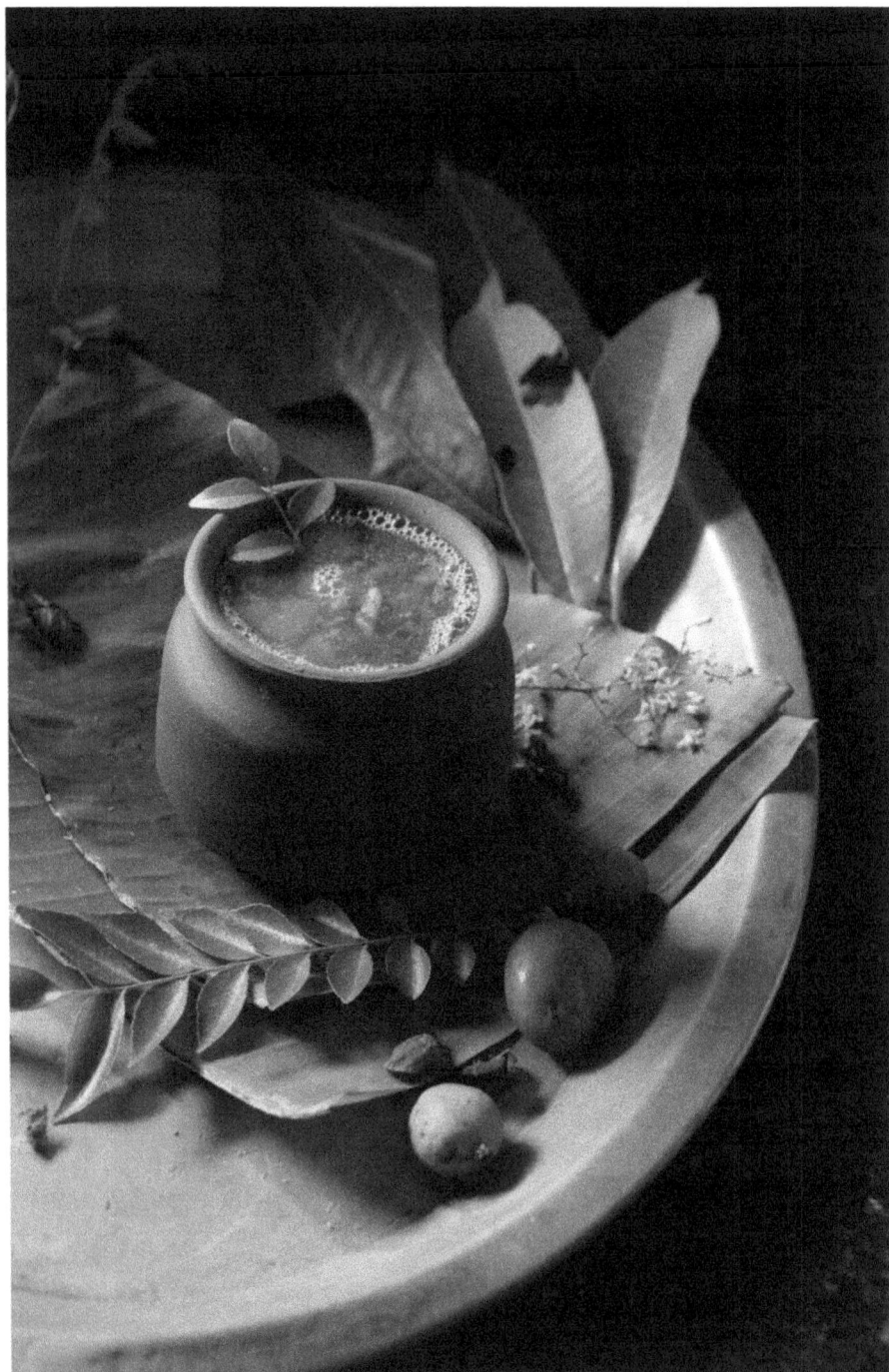

acknowledge that the author is not engaging in the rendering of legal, financial, medical or professional advice. The content within this book has been derived from various sources. Please consult a licensed professional before attempting any techniques outlined in this book.

By reading this document, the reader agrees that under no circumstances is the author responsible for any losses, direct or indirect, which are incurred as a result of the use of information contained within this document, including, but not limited to, — errors, omissions, or inaccuracies.

# Table of Contents

RED LENTILS WITH SPINACH ............................................. 8

VEGETARIAN BALLS IN GRAVY ........................................ 10

QUINOA WITH VEGGIES ....................................................13

QUINOA WITH ASPARAGUS.............................................16

QUINOA & BEANS WITH VEGGIES...................................18

COCONUT BROWN RICE ................................................. 20

BROWN RICE & CHERRIES PILAF ................................... 22

BROWN RICE CASSEROLE............................................... 24

RICE, LENTILS & VEGGIE CASSEROLE .......................... 26

HERBED BULGUR PILAF................................................... 29

ZOODLES...........................................................................31

BIRYANI ........................................................................... 33

GREEK MIXED ROASTED VEGETABLES.......................... 35

AUTUMN ROASTED GREEN BEANS ............................... 38

ROASTED SUMMER SQUASH...........................................40

SAVORY BAKED ACORN SQUASH ..................................41

ROASTED BRUSSELS SPROUTS....................................... 42

ROASTED ROSEMARY POTATOES ................................. 44

SWEET POTATO WEDGES ............................................... 47

BEST LENTIL CURRY ...................................................... 48

CHANA MASALA ............................................................. 50

ZUCCHINI NOODLE PASTA WITH AVOCADO PESTO ......... 52

THAI SOUP ................................................... 54

VEGAN LASAGNA.............................................. 56

CAPRESE ZOODLES............................................ 58

BURRITO ZOODLES ........................................... 59

RED PEPPER ZOODLES ........................................61

ZOODLES MARINARA .................................... 62

ZOODLE JAPCHAE ........................................ 64

BRAISED COLLARDS WITH DRY WINE ........................... 66

CURRY CAULIFLOWER.......................................... 67

GRUEL WITH COCONUT AND SEEDS ............................. 69

BREAKFAST RASPBERRY AND WALNUT CEREAL ............. 70

KETO LASAGNA WITH CASHEW-SPINACH SOUR CREAM . 72

YUMMY FAMILY TACOS .........................................75

MEDLEY WITH SPINACH AND CAULIFLOWER.................. 78

BREAKFAST GRANOLA WITH A TWIST............................80

KETO "TAGLIATELLE" WITH ALMOND BUTTER.............. 82

HOLIDAY ONE-POT-WONDER.................................. 83

VEGAN KETO SOUP .......................................... 85

CREAMY CHOWDER WITH ASPARAGUS AND MUSHROOM 87

MUSHROOM DELIGHT WITH BARBECUE SAUCE ............ 89

MEDITERRANEAN ZOODLES WITH AVOCADO ..................91

CHINESE VEGAN STEW........................................ 93

CHUNKY AUTUMN CHOWDER ................................. 95

CHOWDER WITH ZUCCHINI AND LEEK ........................... 97

BAKED LAMB STEW ........................................................ 99

HADDOCK & POTATO STEW ......................................... 101

ADZUKI BEANS & CARROT STEW ................................. 103

BLACK-EYED BEANS STEW ........................................... 105

# Red Lentils with Spinach

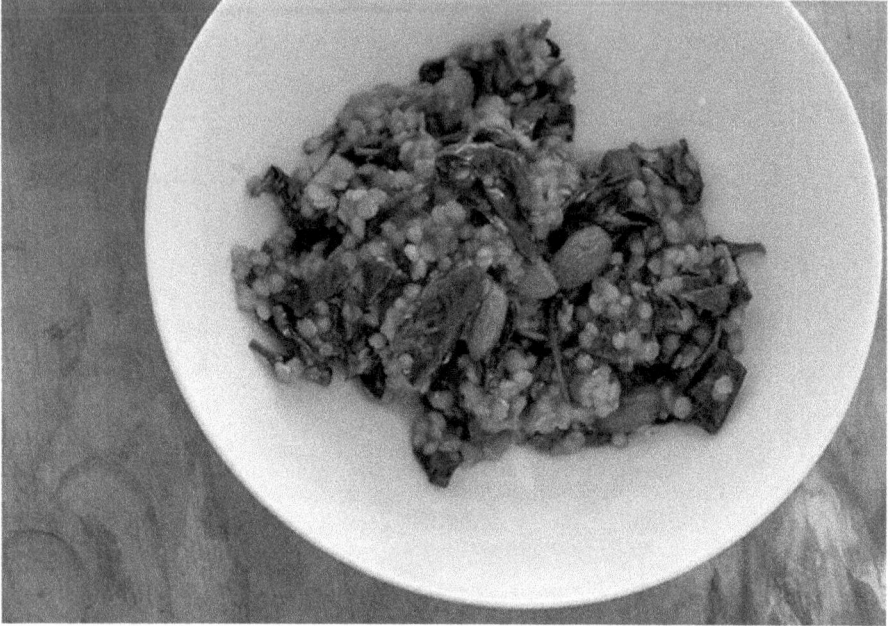

**Prep Time:** 15 min | **Cook Time:** 30 min | **Serve:** 4

- 3½ cups water
- 1½ cups red lentils, soaked for 20 minutes and drained
- ½ teaspoon red chili powder
- ½ teaspoon ground turmeric
- Salt, to taste
- 1-pound fresh spinach, chopped
- 2 tablespoons coconut oil

- 1 onion, chopped
- 1 teaspoon mustard seeds
- 1 teaspoon ground cumin
- ½ cup coconut milk
- 1 teaspoon garam masala

1.In a large pan, add water, lentils, red chili powder, turmeric and salt and bring to a boil on high heat.

2.Reduce the heat to low and simmer, covered for about 15 minutes.

3.Stir in spinach and simmer for about 5 minutes.

4.In a frying pan, melt coconut oil on medium heat.

5.Add onion, mustard seeds and cumin and sauté for about 4-5 minutes.

6.Transfer the onion mixture into the pan with the lentils and stir to combine.

7.Stir in coconut milk and garam masala and simmer for about 3-4 minutes.

**Nutrition:** Calories: 362, Fat: 14g, Sat Fat: 2g, Carbohydrates: 49g, Fiber: 13g, Sugar: 5g, Protein: 21g, Sodium: 693mg

# Vegetarian Balls in Gravy

**Prep Time:** 20 min | **Cook Time:** 25 min | **Serve:** 4-6

For Balls:

- 1 cup cooked chickpeas
- 1 cup cooked red kidney beans
- ½ cup cooked quinoa
- Salt and freshly ground black pepper, to taste 2 tablespoons black beans flour 1 medium onion, chopped
- 2 garlic cloves, chopped
- ¼ cup fresh cilantro, chopped
- 1 teaspoon cumin seeds
- Pinch of baking soda
- 1 tablespoon fresh lemon juice
- 2 teaspoons olive oil

For Gravy:

- 1 teaspoon olive oil
- 1 teaspoon cumin seeds
- 1 medium onion, chopped finely

- 1 (1-inch) piece fresh ginger, grated finely
- 2 tomatoes, chopped finely
- 2 green chilies, chopped finely
- ½ teaspoon garam masala
- ½ teaspoon ground turmeric
- ½ teaspoon red chili powder
- Salt, to taste
- 2 cups water
- ¼ cup fresh cilantro, chopped

1.For balls in a food processor, add all ingredients except oil and pulse till a coarse meal forms.

2.Transfer the mixture into a bowl.

3.Cover the bowl with a foil paper and refrigerate for at least 1 hour.

4.Remove the mixture from refrigerator and make equal sized balls.

5.In a nonstick skillet, heat oil on medium heat.

6.Cook the balls for about 2-3 minutes or till golden brown from all sides.

7.For gravy in a nonstick pan, heat oil on medium heat.

8.Add cumin seeds and sauté for about 1 minute.

9.Add onion and sauté for about 6-7 minutes.

10.Stir in ginger, tomatoes, green chilies and spices and cook for about 1-2 minutes.

11.Add water and bring to a boil.

12.Reduce the heat to low and simmer, covered for about 10 minutes.

13.Carefully, place the balls in the gravy and cook for about 1-2 minutes.

14.Sprinkle with cilantro and serve.

# Quinoa with Veggies

**Prep Time:** 15 min | **Cook Time:** 35 min | **Serve:** 3

- 2 tablespoons olive oil
- 1 small onion, minced
- 2 carrots, peeled and sliced
- 1 celery stalk, chopped
- 1 garlic clove, minced
- ½ cup uncooked quinoa, rinsed
- 1 teaspoon ground turmeric
- ¼ teaspoon dried basil, crushed
- Salt, to taste
- 1 cup vegetable broth
- 1 teaspoon fresh lime juice

1.In a pan, heat oil on medium heat.

2.Add onion, carrot, celery and garlic and sauté for about t minutes.

3.Stir in remaining ingredients except lime juice and bring to a gentle simmer.

4.Reduce the heat to low and simmer, covered for about 25-30 minutes or till all the liquid is absorbed.

5.Stir in lime juice and serve.

**Nutrition:** Calories: 227, Fat: 11g, Sat Fat: 5g, Carbohydrates: 23g, Fiber: 32, Sugar: 2g, Protein: 2g, Sodium: 195mg

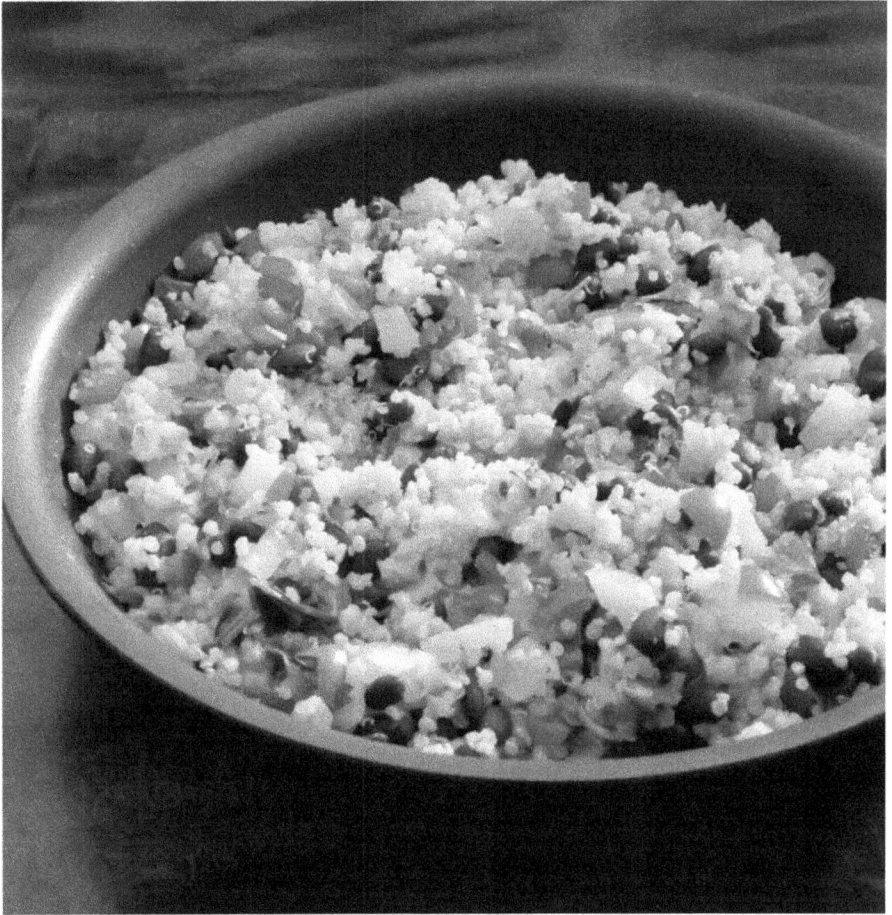

# Quinoa with Asparagus

**Prep Time:** 15 min | **Cook Time:** 18 min | **Serve:** 4

- 1-pound fresh asparagus, trimmed
- 2 teaspoons coconut oil
- ½ of onion, chopped
- 2 minced garlic cloves
- 1 cup cooked red quinoa
- 1 tablespoon ground turmeric
- ½ cup reduced-sodium vegetable broth
- ½ cup nutritional yeast
- 1 tablespoon fresh lemon juice

1.In a large pan of boiling water, cook the asparagus for about 2-3 minutes.

2.Drain well and rinse under cold water.

3.In a large skillet, melt coconut oil on medium heat.

4.Add onion and garlic and sauté for about 5 minutes.

5.Stir in quinoa, turmeric and broth and cook for about 5-6 minutes.

6.Stir in nutritional yeast, lemon juice and asparagus and cook for about 3-4 minutes.

**Nutrition:** Calories: 166, Fat: 2g, Sat Fat: 1g, Carbohydrates: 21g, Fiber: 9g, Sugar: 9g, Protein: 13g, Sodium: 37mg

# Quinoa & Beans with Veggies

**Prep Time:** 20 min | **Cook Time:** 26 min | **Serve:** 6

- 2 cups water
- 1 cup dry quinoa
- 2 tablespoons coconut oil
- 1 medium onion, chopped
- 4 garlic cloves, chopped finely
- 2 tablespoons curry powder
- ½ teaspoon ground turmeric
- Cayenne pepper, to taste
- Salt, to taste
- 2 cups broccoli, chopped
- 1 cup fresh kale, trimmed and chopped
- 1 cup green peas, shelled
- 1 red bell pepper, seeded and chopped
- 2 cups canned kidney beans, rinsed and drained
- 2 tablespoons fresh lime juice

1.In a pan, add water and bring to a boil on high heat.
2.Add quinoa and reduce the heat to low.

3.Simmer for about 10-15 minutes or till all the liquid is absorbed.

4.In a large skillet, melt coconut oil on medium heart.

5.Add onion, garlic, curry powder, turmeric, salt, and sauté for about 4-5 minutes.

6.Add the vegetables and cook for about 5-6 minutes.

7.Stir in quinoa and beans,

8.Drizzle with lime juice and serve.

# Coconut Brown Rice

**Prep Time:** 15 min | **Cook Time:** 1 hour | **Serve:** 14

- 12 cups water
- 1 tablespoon dried turmeric
- 2 pound brown rice
- 2 (13½-ounce) cans lite coconut milk
- 2 (13½-ounce) cans coconut milk
- 1 tablespoon fresh ginger, minced
- 1½ teaspoons fresh lemon zest, grated finely 4 dried bay leaves
- Salt and freshly ground black pepper, to taste Chopped cashews, for garnishing
- Chopped fresh cilantro, for garnishing

1.In a small bowl, add water and turmeric and beat till well combined.

2.In a large pan, add turmeric water and remaining ingredients except cashews and stir well.

3.Bring to a boil on high heat.

4.Reduce the heat to medium and simmer, stirring occasionally for about 30-35 minutes.

5.Reduce the heat to low and simmer, covered for about 20-25 minutes.

6.Remove bay leaf before serving.

7.Garnish with cashews and cilantro and serve.

**Nutrition:** Calories: 184, Fat: 2g, Carbohydrates: 27g, Fiber: 7g, Sugar: 9g, Protein: 2g, Sodium: 76mg,

# Brown Rice & Cherries Pilaf

**Prep Time:** 20 min | **Cook Time:** 35 min | **Serve:** 8

- 1 (14-ounce) can low-sodium vegetable broth 1/3 cup water
- 1 cup brown basmati rice
- 1 tablespoon curry powder
- ½ teaspoon ground turmeric
- Pinch of saffron threads, crumbled
- 1/3 cup fresh lemon juice
- 3 tablespoons olive oil
- 3 tablespoons raw honey
- 1 tablespoon fresh ginger, minced
- 1 tablespoon fresh orange zest, grated finely Salt, to taste
- ¾ cup celery stalk, chopped
- ½ cup scallion, chopped, divided
- ¾ cup dried cherries, chopped roughly
- 1 cup fresh dark sweet cherries, pitted and chopped ¾ cup unsalted mixed nuts

1.In a pan, mix broth, water, rice, curry powder, turmeric and saffron and bring to a boil on medium-high heat.

2.Reduce the heat to low and simmer, covered for about 35 minutes.

3.Remove from heat and keep aside, covered for about 5 minutes.

4.With a fork, fluff the rice.

5.In a large glass bowl, mix lemon juice, oil, honey, ginger, orange zest and salt.

6.Stir in cooked rice, celery, ¼ cup of scallion and dried cherries.

7.Serve immediately with the topping of fresh cherries, nuts and remaining scallion.

**Nutrition:** Calories: 288, Fat: 12g, Sat Fat: 1g, Carbohydrates: 41g, Fiber: 5g, Protein: 6g, Sodium: 125mg

# Brown Rice Casserole

**Prep Time:** 15 min | **Cook Time:** 1 hour | **Serve:** 2

- 1 teaspoon extra-virgin olive oil
- 1 red onion, sliced thinly
- 1½ teaspoons ground turmeric
- 9-ounce brown mushrooms, sliced
- 1 teaspoon raisins
- ½ cup brown rice, rinsed
- 1¼ cups vegetable broth
- ¼ cup fresh cilantro, chopped
- ½ tablespoons pine nuts, toasted
- 1 tablespoon fresh lemon juice
- Salt and freshly ground black pepper, to taste

Preheat the oven to 400 degrees F.

1.In an ovenproof casserole, heat oil on medium heat.

2.Add onion and turmeric and sauté for about 3 minutes.

3.Add mushrooms and stir fry for about 2 minutes.

4.Stir in raisins, rice and broth and transfer into oven.

5.Bake for about 45-55 minutes or till desired doneness.

6.Just before serving, stir in remaining ingredients.

**Nutrition:** Calories: 201, Fat: 5g, Sat Fat: 6g, Carbohydrates: 37g, Fiber: 5g, Sugar: 18g, Protein: 7g, Sodium: 384mg

# Rice, Lentils & Veggie Casserole

**Prep Time:** 20 min | **Cook Time:** 1 h 36 m | **Serve:** 10

- 3¾ cups water, divided
- ½ cup brown lentils, rinsed
- ½ cup wild rice, rinsed
- 1 tbsp olive oil
- ½ of medium onion, chopped
- 1 cup button mushrooms, sliced
- 1 cup tomato sauce
- 1 (10-ounce) package frozen spinach, thawed and squeezed
- 1 (16-ounce) package frozen peas, thawed
- 2 minced garlic cloves
- 1 tablespoon dried oregano, crushed
- 1 teaspoon smoked paprika
- ½ teaspoon ground turmeric
- ¼ cup nutritional yeast

For Sauce

- 1¼ cups unsweetened almond milk
- 1 cup unsalted cashews, soaked for 30 minutes and drained
- 1 teaspoon coconut aminos
- ½ teaspoon dried garlic

1.In a pan, add 3 ½ cups of water, lentils and rice and bring to a boil.

2.Reduce the heat to low and simmer, covered for about 35 minutes.

3.Remove from heat and keep aside to cool.

4.Preheat the oven to 350 degrees F. Grease a 13x9-inch casserole dish.

5.In a large skillet, heat 2 tablespoons of water on high heat.

6.Add onion and sauté for about 2-3 minutes.

7.Add mushrooms and cook for about 2 minutes.

8.Add remaining 2 tablespoons of water and remaining ingredients except nutritional yeast and cook for about 1 minute.

9.Remove from heat and mix with rice mixture.

10.Transfer the mixture into prepared casserole dish evenly.

11.In a blender, add all sauce ingredients and pulse till smooth.

12.Spread the sauce over the rice mixture evenly and stir to combine well.

13.Top with nutritional yeast evenly.

14.Bake for about 45 minutes.

# Herbed Bulgur Pilaf

**Prep Time:** 20 min | **Cook Time:** 35 min | **Serve:** 6

- 2 tablespoons extra-virgin olive oil
- 2 cups onion, chopped
- 1 garlic clove, minced
- 1½ cups medium bulgur
- ½ teaspoon ground cumin
- ½ teaspoon ground turmeric
- 1½ cups carrot, peeled and chopped
- 2 teaspoons fresh ginger, grated finely
- Salt, to taste
- 2 cups vegetable broth
- 3 tablespoons fresh lemon juice
- ¼ cup fresh parsley, chopped
- ¼ cup fresh mint leaves, chopped
- ¼ cup fresh dill, chopped
- ½ cup walnuts, toasted and chopped

1.In a large deep skillet, heat oil on medium-low heat.

2.Add onion and cook, stirring occasionally for about 12-18 minutes.

3.Add garlic and sauté fir about 1 minute.

4.Add bulgur, cumin and turmeric and stir fry for about 1 minute.

5.Add carrot, ginger, salt and broth and bring to a boil, stirring occasionally.

6.Simmer, covered for about 15 minutes.

7.Remove from heat and keep aside, covered for about 5 minutes.

8.Stir in lemon juice and fresh herbs and serve with the garnishing of walnuts.

**Nutrition:** Calories: 277, Fat: 12g, Sat Fat: 1g, Carbohydrates: 39g, Fiber: 10g, Protein: 7g, Sodium: 507mg

# Zoodles

**Prep Time:** 5 min | **Cook Time:** 0 min | **Serve:** 2

- Zucchini 4 organic

Directions- Zoodle Creation

1.If you have access to a spiralizer, use it to create noodles of zucchini. If you do not own a spiralizer, this recipe is still very simple. Just slice the zucchini into long thin strips. You may also wish to use a cheese and vegetable grater to get the desired noodle effect.

2.Serve the zoodles as they are or let them boil for two minutes in a pan of water to warm them up and soften them a bit. Alternately, you may wish to sauté them in a bit of coconut oil or Coconut oil for a minute or two to give them a little crispness.

3.Serve the zoodles in place of the traditional noodles in your favorite pasta dishes.

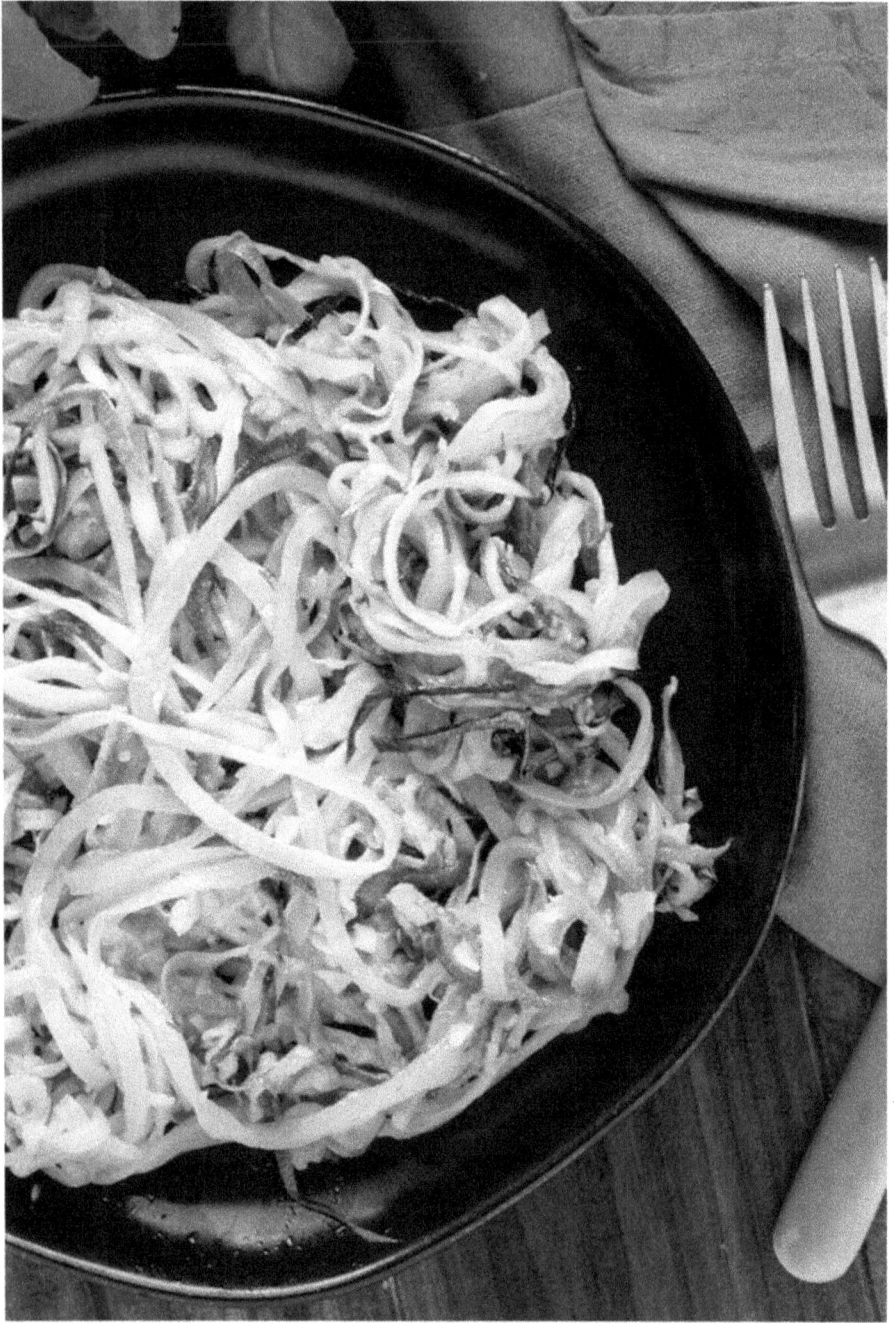

# Biryani

**Prep Time:** 15 min | **Cook Time:** 15 min | **Serve:** 6

- Black pepper as desired
- Sea salt as desired
- Garam masala .5 tsp
- Coconut oil 1 tsp
- Shelled peas 1 c
- Water 5 c
- Coriander .5 tsp ground
- Chili powder 1 tsp
- Turmeric 5 tsp
- Carrots 2 quartered
- Potatoes 2 quartered
- Bay leaves 2 torn
- Cumin seeds .5 tsp
- Onion 1 sliced thin
- Vegetable oil 3 T
- White rice long grain 2 c

1.Add the rice to a large pot and cover it with three to four inches of water before allowing it to soak for about 20 minutes. Drain and set aside.

2.Add the oil to your pressure cooker and set it over medium heat. Add in the onion, bay leaves, and cumin seeds and let everything cook about 5 minutes until the onion is nearly see through.

3.Mix in the carrots and potatoes and cook an additional 5 minutes and the potatoes have begun to brown. Add in the coriander, turmeric and chili powder and let everything cook 1 additional minute.

4.Add the rice to the pressure cooker and ensure it is well covered in the boil before adding peas and water. Mix in the garam masala, oil, and salt before sealing the cooker and turning it to high pressure. Let everything cook for 5 minutes before removing from heat.

5.Allow the pressure to naturally release and fluff the rice with a fork before serving.

# Greek Mixed Roasted Vegetables

**Prep Time:** 15 min | **Cook Time:** 45 min | **Serve:** 4

Ingredients- Vegetables

- 1 eggplant peeled and diced .75-inch
- Black pepper as desired
- Kosher sea salt as desired
- Extra virgin olive oil 2 T
- Garlic 2 cloves minced
- Onion 1 peeled, diced 1-inch
- Bell pepper 2 red, yellow, diced, 1-inch

Ingredients- Dressing

- Coconut oil .25 c
- Lemon juice .3 c squeezed fresh
- Black pepper as desired
- Kosher sea salt as desired
- Basil 15 leaves
- Scallions 4 minced

1.Ensure your oven is heated to 425F.

2.One a sheet pan, combine the garlic, onion, yellow bell pepper, red bell pepper, and eggplant before seasoning using the pepper, salt, and coconut oil.

3.Add the pan to the oven and let it cook for 40 minutes, using a spatula to flip everything after 20 minutes.

4.As the vegetables are cooking, combine the pepper, salt, coconut oil, and lemon juice in a small bowl and add the vegetables' results as soon as they are ready.

5.Let the pan cool completely before adding in the basil, feta, and scallions. Season before serving.

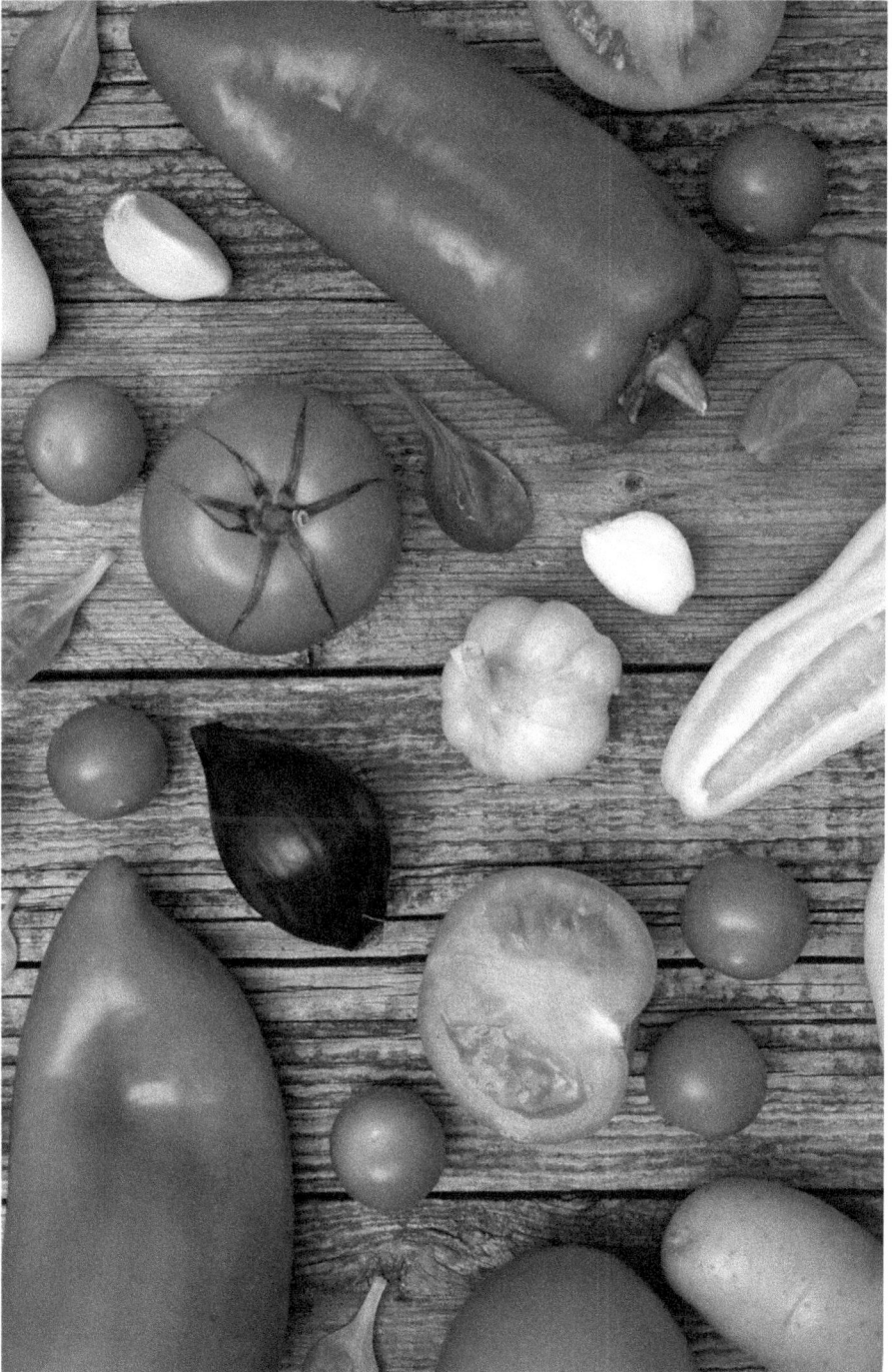

# Autumn Roasted Green Beans

**Prep Time:** 15 min | **Cook Time:** 30 min | **Serve:** 4

- Walnuts .5 c toasted
- Cranberries .5 c dried
- Black pepper as desired
- Kosher sea salt as desired
- Lemon juice 2 tsp.
- Lemon zest 1 tsp.
- Sugar .25 tsp.
- Coconut oil 2 T
- Garlic 4 cloves, quartered and peeled
- Green beans 2 lbs. stems trimmed

1.Preheat your oven to 350F and crack and smash the walnuts into chunks.

2.Spread the walnuts onto a baking sheet and toast them for 10 minutes.

3.Increase the temperature on the oven to 450F.

4.Cover a baking sheet with a rim using aluminum foil.

5.In a mixing bowl, combine the sugar, pepper, salt, and coconut oil before thoroughly coating the garlic and green beans.

6.Place the beans onto a baking sheet and spread them out to ensure they cook well. Place the sheet into the oven and let the beans bake for 15 minutes, before stirring with a spatula and roasting another 10 minutes.

7.Mix in the lemon juice, pepper and salt before serving.

# Roasted Summer Squash

**Prep Time:** 5 min | **Cook Time:** 30 min | **Serve:** 4

- Zucchini 3
- Yellow squash 3
- Kosher salt 5 T
- Black pepper .5 T
- Coconut oil 2 T

1.Ensure your oven is heated to 400F

2.Peel vegetables and cut into.25 inch thick slices.

3.Assemble vegetables on a baking sheet or pan and drizzle coconut oil on top. Sprinkle with seasoning as desired

4.Bake at 400F for 30 minutes.

# Savory Baked Acorn Squash

**Prep Time:** 5 min | **Cook Time:** 30 min | **Serve:** 4

- Acorn squash 1
- Kosher salt as desired
- Black pepper as desired
- Coconut oil 2 tsp.
- Smoked paprika as desired

1.Ensure your oven is heated to 425F.

2.Cut acorn squash in half lengthwise, then cut halves into quarters lengthwise. Scoop out seeds and discard.

3.Place the squash on baking sheet and drizzle coconut oil over the top of each quarter. Scatter with the smoked paprika, salt, and pepper and bake in the oven for 30 minutes.

# Roasted Brussels Sprouts

**Prep Time:** 5 min | **Cook Time:** 15 min | **Serve:** 4

- Sea salt .25 tsp.
- Black pepper .25 tsp.
- Brussel sprouts .75lbs. sliced in half length-wise
- Coconut oil 5 T.

1.Ensure your oven is heated to 400F. Cut Brussels sprouts in half and place in a medium-sized bowl. Drizzle the coconut oil over the Brussels sprouts and then toss with the sea salt and black pepper until evenly coated.

2.Pour Brussels sprouts onto a baking sheet and make sure they are evenly spaced so that they will roast easily.

3.Place the sheet in the oven and let it cook approximately 10 minutes before stirring well and returning it to the oven for 10 minutes more. Season as desired They will keep in the fridge for 3-4 days, or in the freezer for 2-3 months.

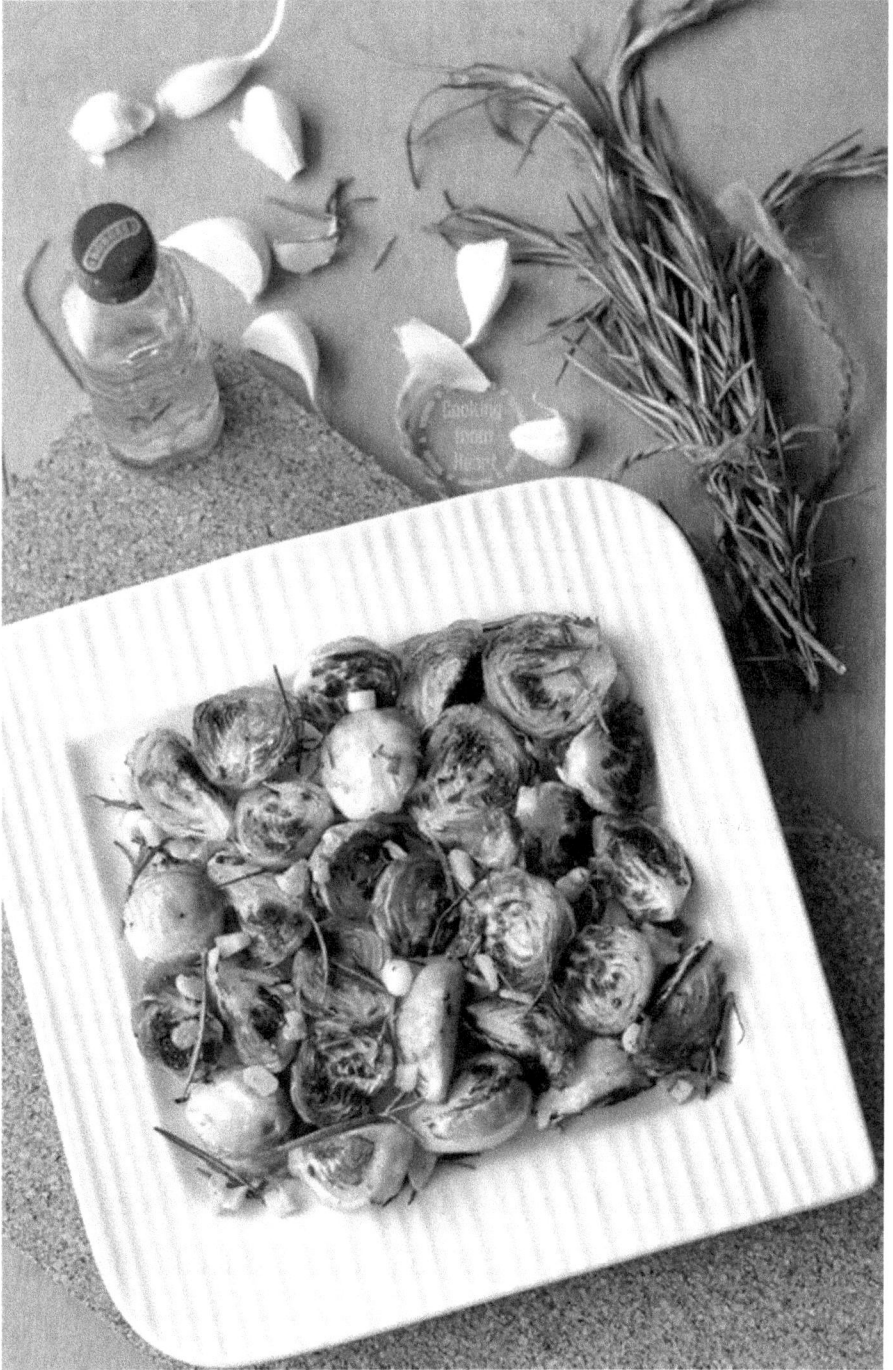

# Roasted Rosemary Potatoes

**Prep Time:** 10 min | **Cook Time:** 25 min | **Serve:** 6

- Garlic 1 head
- Rosemary 3 sprigs
- Thyme 3 sprigs
- Baby potatoes 20 oz.
- Parsley 2 T chopped
- Sea salt as desired
- Black pepper as desired
- Coconut oil 2 T

1.Ensure your oven is heated to 450F.

2.Separate garlic cloves and remove the papery skin holding them together, but do not peel.

3.Add the rosemary, thyme, baby potatoes, parsley, garlic, and coconut oil together in a large bowl, coating well.

4.Add the results to a jelly roll pan that has been lined with tinfoil before topping with pepper and salt. Place the pan in the oven and let the potatoes bake approximately 25 minutes, stirring at the 12-minute mark.

5.Season with additional pepper and salt before serving.

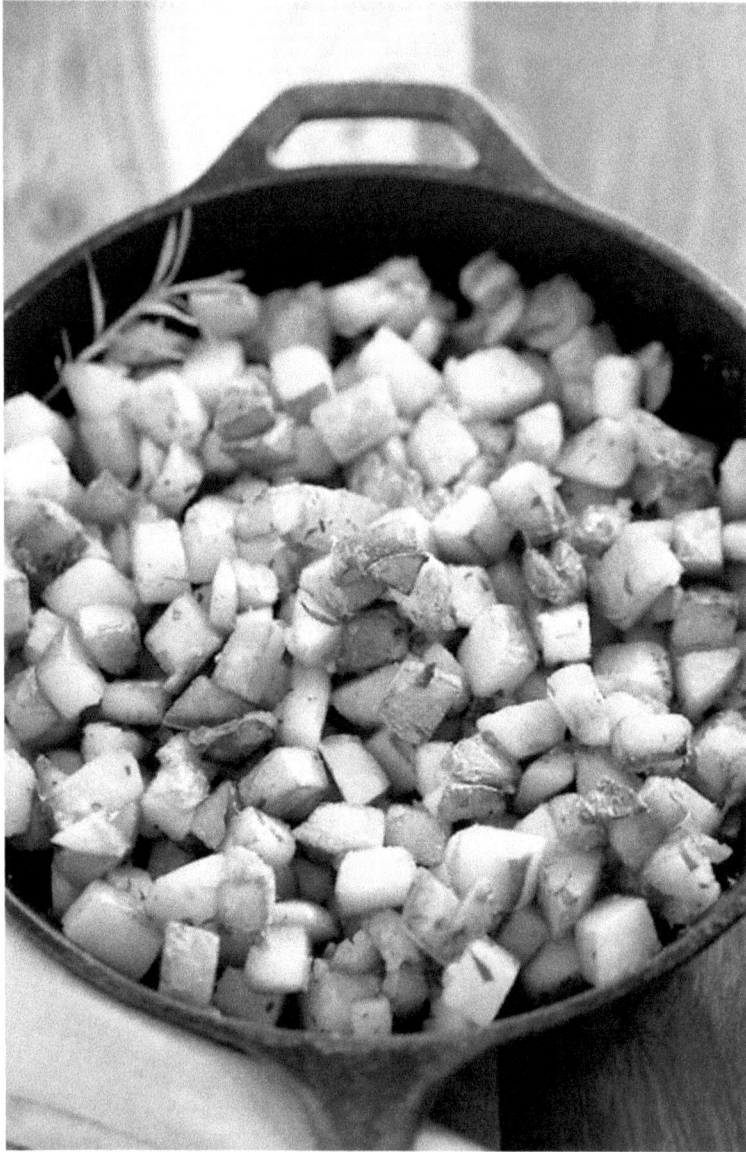

# Sweet Potato Wedges

**Prep Time:** 10 min | **Cook Time:** 30 min | **Serve:** 6

- Salt 1 tsp.
- Cracked black pepper 1 tsp.
- Garlic powder .5 tsp.
- Sweet potatoes 4 medium, peeled, each cut into 6 wedges
- Rosemary 1 T chopped, fresh
- Coconut oil 2 T

1.Preheat oven to 450F.

2.In a mixing bowl, combine the coconut oil, rosemary, sweet potatoes, garlic powder, black pepper, and salt and ensure the potatoes are coated well.

3.Add the results in a single layer to a large roasting pan before placing the pan in the oven and letting the potatoes bake for 20 minutes. Turn the dish at this point before baking another 10 minutes.

# Best Lentil Curry

**Prep Time:** 10 min | **Cook Time:** 30 min | **Serve:** 4

- Vegetable broth 4 c low sodium
- Red lentil 1 c
- Potato 10 oz. peeled and made into pieces that are 1 inch each
- Carrot 8 oz. chopped
- Curry powder 1 T
- Scallions 8 separated, sliced
- Garlic 2 cloves chopped
- Ginger 2 T chopped
- Coconut oil 3 T

1.Add the oil to a saucepan before placing it on the stove on top of a burner set to a high/medium heat.

2.Add in the scallion whites, garlic and ginger and let them soften for 2 minutes.

3.Mix in the curry powder and pepper and salt, as desired, broth, lentils, potato, and carrots before letting everything boil. Turn down the heat and let everything simmer for 15 minutes, stirring regularly.

4.Top with scallion greens before serving.

# Chana Masala

**Prep Time:** 5 min | **Cook Time:** 25 min | **Serve:** 4

- Curry powder 1 tsp.
- Chickpeas 32 oz. rinsed, drained
- Garlic 2 cloves minced
- Onion 1 large, chopped
- Extra virgin olive oil 1 T
- Cilantro .25 c
- Kosher sea salt as desired
- Lemon juice 1 T
- Tomatoes 2 chopped
- Ginger 2 tsp. grated
- Turmeric .5 tsp.

1.Add the oil to a skillet before placing it on a burner set to a medium/high heat. Add in the onion and let it sauté until it has become translucent and soft. Mix in the garlic and let it cook for 3 minutes.

2.Add in the curry powder, chickpeas, coconut oil, lemon juice, tomatoes, ginger and turmeric along with.25 c of water. Let the mixture simmer before cooking it for 10 minutes, stirring on occasion. The result should have a stew-like consistency but not be runny.

3.Season using salt and top with cilantro before serving.

# Zucchini Noodle Pasta with Avocado Pesto

**Prep Time:** 30 min | **Cook Time:** 15 min | **Serve:** 8

- Zucchinis 6 spiralized
- Cold pressed oil of choice 1 T

Ingredients- Pesto

- Pine nuts .25 c
- Avocados 2 cubed
- Parsley .25 c leaves
- Basil 1 c leaves
- Garlic 3 cloves
- Lemon juice 1 lemon
- Cold pressed oil of choice 3 T
- Salt as desired
- Pepper as desired

1.Spiralize your zucchini and set aside on paper towels.

2.In a food processor, add in all ingredients for the avocado pesto except the oil. Pulse on low until desired consistency is reached.

3.Slowly add in coconut oil until creamy and emulsified.

4.Heat 1 T and your zucchini noodles cook for 4 min.

5.Take your zucchini noodles and coat with avocado pesto.

# Thai Soup

**Prep Time:** 30 min | **Cook Time:** 15 min | **Serve:** 9

- Spiralized Zucchinis 2 medium
- Minced Garlic Cloves 2 total
- Thin Sliced Red Pepper 1 total
- Diced Jalapeno 1 total
- Lime 1 cut into 8 wedges
- Thin Sliced Onion 5 total
- Full-Fat Coconut Milk 15oz
- Vegetable Broth 6 c
- Fresh Chopped Cilantro 5 c
- Green Curry Paste 5 T
- Coconut Oil 1 T

1.Add the coconut oil to a saucepan before adding in the onions and letting them sauté. Takes about 5 minutes.

2.Add jalapeno, curry paste, and minced garlic. Sauté for 1 minute or until just fragrant. Stir in bone broth and coconut milk, mix until thoroughly combined. Heat until soup comes to a boil and then reduce to medium heat. Add red pepper slices, then mix.

3.Simmer soup approximately 5 minutes or until done, until chicken is cooked through. Add fresh cilantro.

4.Divide zucchini into 8 bowls and ladle soup over them. The heat of the soup will cook the zucchini noodles. If not serving all at once, store soup and zoodles separately and combine when prepared to eat, so zoodles don't become soggy.

# Vegan Lasagna

**Prep Time:** 10 min | **Cook Time:** 4 hours | **Serve:** 8

- Lasagna Zoodles 6
- Vegan cheese 5 c
- Red pepper flakes .25 tsp.
- Basil .5 tsp. dried
- Oregano 1 tsp. dried
- Salt 1 tsp.
- Tomato sauce 15 oz.
- Tomato 28 oz. crushed
- Garlic 1 clove minced
- Onion 1 chopped
- Ground soy 1 lb.

1.Place a skillet on the stove on top of a burner set to a high/medium heat before adding garlic, onion, and soy and letting the soy brown.

2.Add in the red pepper flakes, basil, oregano, salt, tomato sauce, and crushed tomatoes and let the results simmer 5 minutes.

3.Add.3 of the total sauce from the skillet and add it to the slow cooker. Place 3 Zoodles on top of the sauce, followed by cheese mixture. Create three layers in total.

4.Cover the slow cooker and let it cook on a low heat for 6 hours.

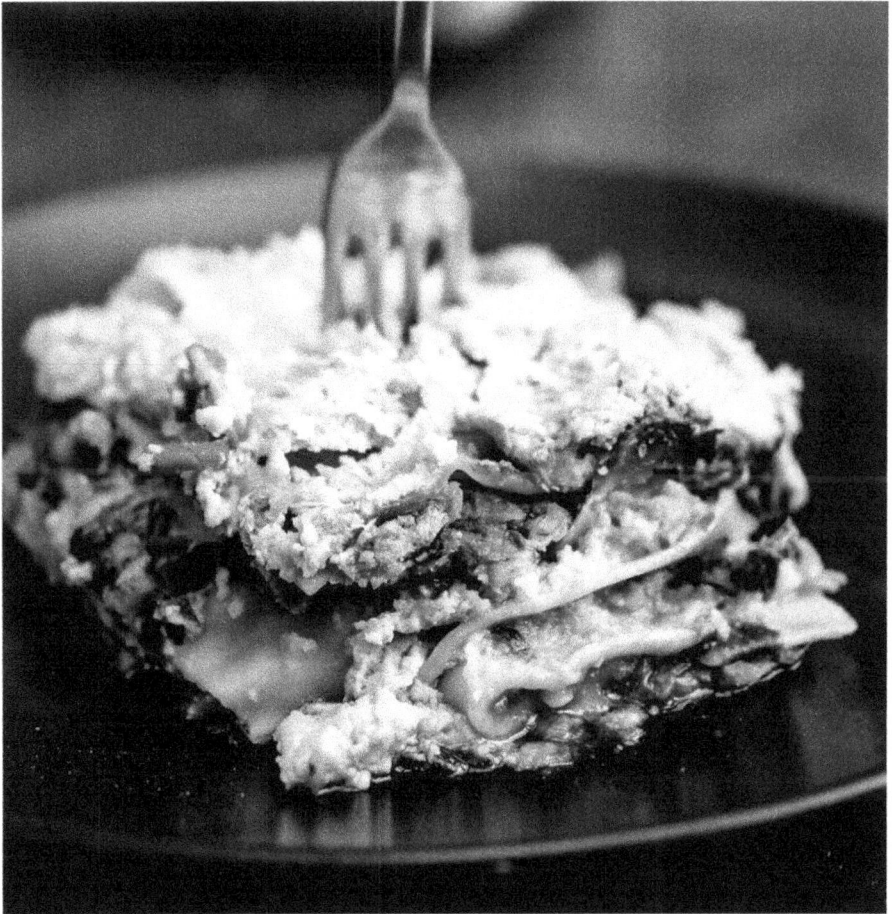

# Caprese Zoodles

**Prep Time:** 10 min | **Cook Time:** 15 min | **Serve:** 4

- Zucchini 4 large
- 2 T coconut oil
- Kosher salt as desired
- Black pepper as desired
- Cherry tomatoes, 2 c halved
- Mozzarella balls 1 c quartered
- Basil leaves .25 c torn
- Balsamic vinegar 2 T

1.Place the zoodles in a serving bowl before adding in the coconut oil and tossing well. Season as desired and allow the zoodles to marinate for at least 15 minutes.

2.Mix in the basil, mozzarella, and tomatoes and toss well.

3.Top with balsamic before serving.

# Burrito Zoodles

**Prep Time:** 25 min | **Cook Time:** 15 min | **Serve:** 4

- Coconut oil 2 T
- Onion 1 medium, chopped
- Garlic 2 cloves minced
- Chili powder 1 tsp.
- Cumin .5 tsp. ground
- Kosher salt as desired
- Black pepperas desired
- Black beans 15 oz. drained and rinsed
- Cherry tomatoes 1 c halved
- Red enchilada sauce 1 c
- Cheddar 1 c shredded
- Monterey Jack 1 c shredded
- Zoodles 14 oz.

1.Add the oil to the skillet before placing it on the stove over a burner turned to medium heat.

2.Add in the carrot and onion and allow both to cook approximately 5 minutes before adding in the garlic and allowing it to cook approximately 60 seconds.

3.Mix in the cumin, chili powder, salt, and pepper before adding in the cheese, enchilada sauce, cherry tomatoes, and black beans.

4.Allow everything to simmer approximately 10 minutes before adding in the zoodles and tossing to coat. Let the zoodles cook approximately 3 minutes, stirring regularly.

# Red Pepper Zoodles

**Prep Time:** 10 min | **Cook Time:** 25 min | **Serve:** 4

- Red bell peppers 1
- Almond milk 1 c
- Coconut oil 1 T
- Salt 1 tsp.
- Garlic 1 clove
- Almond Coconut oil .25 c

1.Prepare a baking sheet by lining it with foil.

2.Add the bell peppers to the baking sheet before placing them on the top level of your broiler and letting them cook until blackened.

3.Once they have cooled you can remove the skins, stems, seeds, and ribs.

4.Add the results, along with the remaining sauce ingredients and blend thoroughly. Season as desired.

5.Serve with zoodles and a variety of potential toppings, including truffle oil, goat cheese, parmesan cheese, or parsley.

# Zoodles Marinara

**Prep Time:** 15 min | **Cook Time:** 15 min | **Serve:** 4

- Extra virgin coconut oil 2 T
- White onions .5 c diced
- Garlic cloves 6 minced
- Tomatoes 14 oz. diced
- Tomato paste 2 T
- Basil leaves .5 c roughly-chopped loosely packed
- Coarse salt 5 tsp
- Black pepper .25 tsp
- Cayenne 1 pinch
- Zucchinis 2 large spiralized
- Parmesan cheese as desired

1.Add the oil to the skillet before placing it on the stove over a burner turned to a medium heat.

2.Add in the onion and allow it to cook approximately 5 minutes before adding in the garlic and allowing it to cook approximately 60 seconds.

3.Mix in the crushed red pepper flakes, pepper, salt, basil tomato paste, and tomatoes and combine thoroughly.

4.Allow the sauce to simmer before reducing the heat to medium/low. Let the sauce simmer an additional 15 minutes or until the oil takes on a deep orange color, which indicates the sauce is thickened and reduced. Season as desired.

5.Add in the zoodles and let them soften approximately 2 minutes.

6.Top with parmesan cheese before serving.

# Zoodle Japchae

**Prep Time:** 15 min | **Cook Time:** 8 min | **Serve:** 2

- Spinach 5 c packed
- Coconut oil 1 T
- Carrot 1 halved
- White onion .5 sliced thin
- Shitake mushrooms 5 oz. sliced
- Zucchini 1 sliced
- Sesame oil 1 T
- Honey 2 tsp.
- Soy sauce 2 T

1.Fill a small pot with water before placing it on the stove over a burner turned to high heat.

2.While waiting for the pot to boil, combine the soy sauce, honey, sesame oil in a small bowl, whisk well and set to one side.

3.After the water, boils add in the spinach and cook until it begins to wilt. Remove it from the water with the help of a slotted spoon and squeeze out any excess water.

4.Add the oil to the skillet before placing it on the stove over a burner turned to medium heat.

5.Add in the onion, carrot and shitake mushrooms before allowing them to cook approximately 5 minutes.

6.Add in the zoodles and toss approximately 2 minutes. Add the results to a colander and toss to remove excess moisture.

7.Return the zoodles to the skillet, add in the spinach and top with the sauce. Toss for approximately 60 seconds.

# Braised Collards with Dry Wine

**Prep Time:** 10 minutes | **Serve:** 4

- 1 pound Collards, torn into pieces
- 1 ½ tablespoons sesame oil
- 1 teaspoon ginger-garlic paste
- Sea salt and ground black pepper, to taste 1/2 teaspoon mustard seeds 1/2 teaspoon fennel seeds
- 3/4 cup water
- 1/4 cup dry red wine

1.Simply throw all of the above ingredients into your Instant Pot.

2.Secure the lid. Choose "Manual" mode and High pressure; cook for 2 minutes. Once cooking is complete, use a quick pressure release; carefully remove the lid.

3.Ladle into individual bowls and serve warm. Bon appétit!

**Nutrition:** 91 Calories; 9g Fat; 7g Total Carbs; 7g, Protein; 1g Sugars

# Curry Cauliflower

**Prep Time:** 10 minutes | **Serve:** 4

- 2 tablespoons grapeseed oil
- ½ cup scallions, chopped
- 2 cloves garlic, pressed
- 1 tablespoon garam masala
- 1 teaspoon curry powder
- 1 red chili pepper, minced
- ½ teaspoon ground cumin
- Sea salt and ground black pepper, to taste 1 tablespoon fresh coriander, chopped 1 teaspoon ajwain
- 2 tomatoes, puréed
- 1 pound cauliflower, broken into florets 1/2 cup water
- ½ cup almond yogurt

1.Press the "Sauté" button to heat your Instant Pot. Now, heat the oil and sauté the scallions for 1 minute.

2.Add garlic and continue to cook an additional 30 seconds or until aromatic.

3.Add garam masala, curry powder, chili pepper, cumin, salt, black pepper, coriander, ajwain, tomatoes, cauliflower, and water.

4.Secure the lid. Choose "Manual" mode and High pressure; cook for 3 minutes. Once cooking is complete, use a quick pressure release; carefully remove the lid.

5.Pour in the almond yogurt, stir well and serve warm.

**Nutrition:** 101 Calories; 2g Fat; 6g Total Carbs; 3g, Protein; 36g Sugars

# Gruel with Coconut and Seeds

**Prep Time:** 10 minutes | **Serve:** 4

- 4 tablespoons shredded coconut, unsweetened
- 2 tablespoons pumpkin seeds
- 2 tablespoons flaxseed
- ½ cup almonds, chopped
- ½ teaspoon grated nutmeg
- ¼ teaspoon ground cloves
- 1 teaspoon ground cinnamon
- Himalayan salt, to taste
- 1 cup boiling water

1.Add all ingredients to the Instant Pot.

2.Secure the lid. Choose "Manual" mode and High pressure; cook for 5 minutes. Once cooking is complete, use a quick pressure release; carefully remove the lid.

3.Serve garnished with some extra slivered almonds if desired.

**Nutrition:** 116 Calories; 15g Fat; 4g Total Carbs; 7g, Protein; 8g Sugars

# Breakfast Raspberry and Walnut Cereal

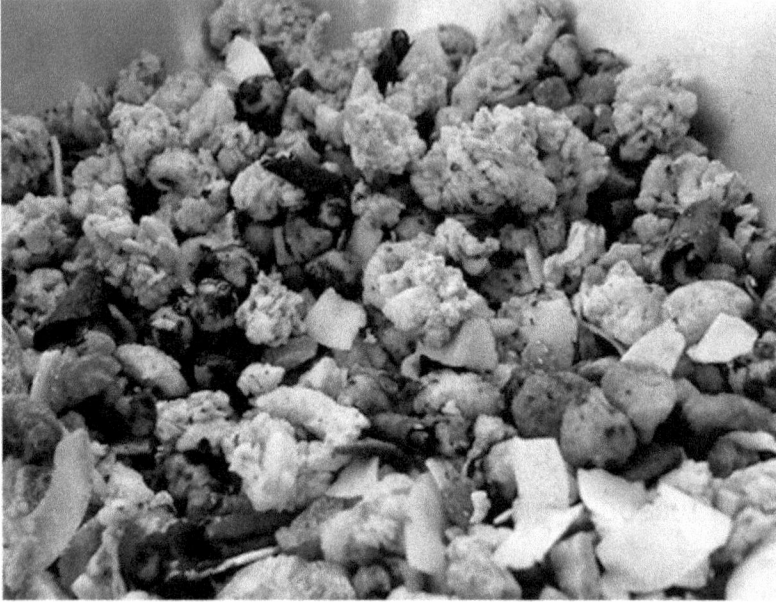

**Prep Time:** 2 hours 10 minutes | **Serve:** 4

- 3/4 cup walnuts, soaked overnight and chopped
- Himalayan salt, to taste
- ¾ cup water
- 2 tablespoons coconut oil
- 1 tablespoon sunflower seeds
- ½ cup dried raspberries
- ½ teaspoon vanilla paste
- ¼ teaspoon star anise, ground

- ¼ teaspoon grated nutmeg
- ½ teaspoon ground cinnamon

1.Add all ingredients to your Instant Pot.

2.Secure the lid. Choose "Slow Cook" mode and High pressure; cook for 2 hours. Once cooking is complete, use a quick pressure release; carefully remove the lid.

3.Spoon into individual bowls and serve warm. Bon appétit!

**Nutrition:** 199 Calories; 17g Fat; 7g Total Carbs; 1g, Protein; 9g Sugars

# Keto Lasagna with Cashew-Spinach Sour Cream

**Prep Time:** 1 hour 20 minutes | **Serve:** 4

Herbed Tomato Sauce:

- 2 teaspoons olive oil
- ½ cup green onions, chopped
- 1 garlic clove, minced
- 2 ripe tomatoes, crushed
- ½ cup water
- 1/2 teaspoon dried rosemary
- 1/2 teaspoon dried basil
- Sea salt and ground black pepper, to taste 1/2 teaspoon cayenne pepper

Cashew-Spinach Sour Cream:

- ½ cup cashews, soaked
- 1 cup water
- 1 cup spinach leaves, torn into pieces
- 2 garlic cloves
- Sea salt and ground black pepper, to taste

Zoodles:

- 4 zucchinis, sliced
- 1 tablespoon salt
- 1/2 teaspoon dried dill
- 2 tablespoons olive oil

1.Press the "Sauté" button to heat your Instant Pot. Now, heat 2 teaspoons of olive oil and sauté the green onions and garlic approximately 2 minutes.

2.Add the tomatoes, water, rosemary, basil, salt, black pepper, and cayenne pepper. Cook until thoroughly heated or approximately 5 minutes.

3.Mix cashews, water, spinach, garlic, salt, and black pepper until everything is well incorporated; reserve.

4.Slice zucchinis and add 1 tablespoon of salt. Let it sit for 30 minutes; drain your zucchinis and season them with dried dill. Now, place 1/2 of zucchini slices on the bottom of a lightly greased casserole dish.

5.Drizzle with 1 tablespoon of olive oil.

6.Add the prepared tomato sauce. Add the remaining 1/2 zucchini slices. Drizzle with 1 tablespoon of olive oil. Top with Cashew-Spinach Sour Cream.

7.Cover the casserole dish with a piece of foil.

8.Secure the lid. Choose "Bean/Chili" mode and High pressure; cook for 25 minutes. Once cooking is complete, use a quick pressure release; carefully remove the lid.

9.Allow this lasagna to cool for 10 to 15 minutes until slicing and serving. Serve warm.

**Nutrition:** 170 Calories; 17g Fat; 6g Total Carbs; 5g, Protein; 7g Sugars

# Yummy Family Tacos

**Prep Time:** 45 minutes | **Serve:** 4

- 1 cup water
- 1 teaspoon ginger-garlic paste
- 2 tablespoons tamari sauce
- 1/4 cup dry white wine

Salt and pepper, to taste

- ½ teaspoon turmeric powder
- 1 teaspoon hot sauce
- 14 ounces extra-firm tofu, pressed and cubed
- 2 tablespoons olive oil
- 1 cup cherry tomatoes, halved
- 1 tablespoon Dijon mustard
- 1 bell pepper, seeded and chopped
- 1 red chili pepper, seeded and minced

Vegan Keto Tortillas:

- 2 tablespoons psyllium husks
- 1 cup almond flour
- ¼ teaspoon baking soda

- ¼ teaspoon baking powder
- Sea salt, to taste
- 2 tablespoons coconut oil, softened
- Hot water, as needed

1.In a mixing dish, combine water, ginger-garlic paste, tamari sauce, wine, salt, pepper, turmeric powder, and hot sauce; add tofu and let it marinate for 30 minutes.

2.Press the "Sauté" button to heat your Instant Pot. Heat the olive oil and brown tofu for 1 to 2 minutes per side.

3.Add the marinade. Secure the lid. Choose "Manual" mode and High pressure; cook for 6 minutes. Once cooking is complete, use a quick pressure release; carefully remove the lid.

4.Thoroughly combine dry ingredients for vegan keto tortillas; add coconut oil and mix again. Now, pour in hot water to form a dough.

5.Divide dough into 4 balls. Flatten each ball into tortilla shapes.

6.Afterwards, grill your tortillas at 350 degrees F until slightly browned on each side.

7.Assemble your tortillas with the prepared tofu, cherry tomatoes, mustard, bell pepper and chili pepper.

**Nutrition:** 251 Calories; 22g Fat; 7g Total Carbs; 13g, Protein; 1g Sugars

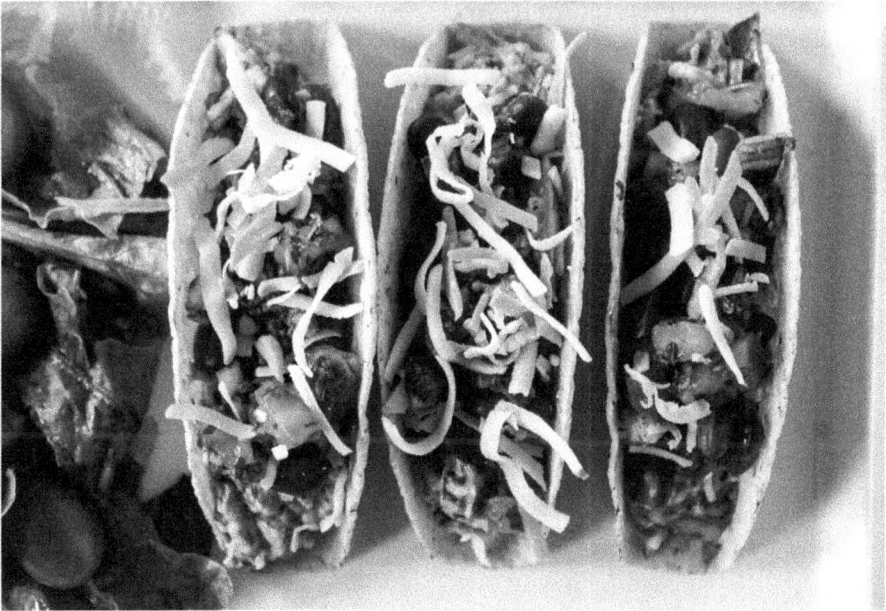

# Medley with Spinach and Cauliflower

**Prep Time:** 10 minutes | **Serve:** 4

- 1 pound cauliflower, broken into florets
- 2 tablespoons olive oil
- 2 garlic cloves, crushed
- 1 yellow onion, peeled and chopped
- 1 celery stalk, chopped
- 1 red bell pepper, seeded and chopped Sea salt and ground black pepper, to taste 1 teaspoon Hungarian paprika
- 1 tablespoon grated lemon zest
- 2 cups spinach, torn into pieces

1.Add cauliflower, olive oil, garlic, onion, celery, bell pepper, salt, pepper, paprika, and lemon zest to the Instant Pot.

2.Secure the lid. Choose "Manual" mode and High pressure; cook for 3 minutes. Once cooking is complete, use a quick pressure release; carefully remove the lid.

3.Add spinach and put the lid on the Instant Pot. Let it sit in the residual heat until wilted.

**Nutrition:** 124 Calories; 5g Fat; 7g Total Carbs; 9g, Protein; 4g Sugars

# Breakfast Granola with a Twist

**Prep Time:** 2 hours 35 minutes | **Serve:** 6

- 1 cup almonds
- 1 cup walnuts
- 2 ounces shredded coconut, unsweetened 1/4 cup sunflower seeds 1/4 cup pumpkin seeds
- 1 teaspoon vanilla paste
- 1/2 teaspoon ground cinnamon
- A pinch of kosher salt
- 1/4 teaspoon star anise, ground
- 2 tablespoons dark rum

1.Place all ingredients in your Instant Pot.

2.Secure the lid. Choose "Slow Cook" mode and High pressure; cook for 2 hours 30 minutes. Once cooking is complete, use a quick pressure release; carefully remove the lid.

3.Spoon into individual bowls and serve warm. Bon appétit!

**Nutrition:** 166 Calories; 12g Fat; 4g Total Carbs; 8g, Protein; 9g Sugars

# Keto "Tagliatelle" with Almond Butter

**Prep Time:** 10 minutes | **Serve:** 4

- 2 tablespoons coconut oil
- 1 yellow onion, chopped
- 2 zucchini, julienned
- 1 cup Chinese cabbage, shredded
- 2 garlic cloves, minced
- 2 tablespoons almond butter
- Sea salt and freshly ground black pepper, to taste 1 teaspoon cayenne pepper

1.Press the "Sauté" button to heat your Instant Pot. Heat the coconut oil and sweat the onion for 2 minutes.

2.Add the other ingredients.

3.Secure the lid. Choose "Manual" mode and High pressure; cook for 2 minutes. Once cooking is complete, use a quick pressure release; carefully remove the lid.

# Holiday One-Pot-Wonder

**Prep Time:** 15 minutes | **Serve:** 4

- 10 ounces coconut milk
- 10 ounces vegetable stock
- 1 garlic cloves, minced
- 1 teaspoon fresh ginger root, grated
- 4 tablespoons almond butter
- Sea salt and ground black pepper, to taste 1/2 teaspoon turmeric powder A pinch of grated nutmeg
- ½ teaspoon ground coriander
- 10 ounces pumpkin, cubed
- 1/3 cup leek, white part only, finely sliced

1.Place the milk, stock, garlic, ginger, almond butter, salt, black pepper, turmeric powder, nutmeg, coriander, and pumpkin in your Instant Pot.

2.Secure the lid. Choose "Manual" mode and High pressure; cook for 10 minutes. Once cooking is complete, use a natural pressure release; carefully remove the lid.

3.Now, blend your soup with a stick blender. Ladle your soup into serving bowls and top with leeks. Bon appétit!

**Nutrition:** 157 Calories; 13g Fat; 4g Total Carbs; 4g, Protein; 7g Sugars

# Vegan Keto Soup

**Prep Time:** 15 minutes | **Serve:** 4

- 2 tablespoons olive oil
- 1 shallot, chopped
- 1 celery, diced
- 3 ripe medium-sized tomatoes, puréed
- 4 cups roasted vegetable stock
- 1 teaspoon granulated garlic
- ½ teaspoon rosemary
- ½ teaspoon lemon thyme
- Himalayan salt and ground white pepper, to taste
- 1 bay leaf
- 4-5 whole cloves
- ½ cup almond milk, unsweetened
- 2 heaping tablespoons fresh parsley, roughly chopped

1.Press the "Sauté" button to heat your Instant Pot. Heat the olive oil and sauté the shallot and celery until softened.

2.Now, add tomatoes, stock, garlic, rosemary, lemon thyme, salt, black pepper, bay leaf, cloves, and milk; stir to combine well.

3.Secure the lid. Choose "Manual" mode and High pressure; cook for 8 minutes. Once cooking is complete, use a natural pressure release; carefully remove the lid.

4.Ladle into individual bowls and top each serving with fresh parsley.

**Nutrition:** 136 Calories; 8g Fat; 8g Total Carbs; 2g, Protein; 3g Sugars

# Creamy Chowder with Asparagus and Mushroom

**Prep Time:** 15 minutes | **Serve:** 4

- 2 tablespoons coconut oil
- ½ cup shallots, chopped
- 2 cloves garlic, minced
- 1 pound asparagus, washed, trimmed and chopped
- 4 ounces button mushrooms, sliced
- 4 cups vegetable broth
- 2 tablespoons balsamic vinegar
- Himalayan salt, to taste
- ¼ teaspoon ground black pepper
- ¼ teaspoon paprika
- ¼ cup vegan sour cream

1.Press the "Sauté" button to heat your Instant Pot. Heat the oil and cook the shallots and garlic for 2 to 3 minutes.
2.Add the remaining ingredients, except for sour cream, to the Instant Pot.

3.Secure the lid. Choose "Manual" mode and High pressure; cook for 4 minutes. Once cooking is complete, use a quick pressure release; carefully remove the lid.

4.Spoon into four soup bowls; add a dollop of sour cream to each serving and serve immediately. Bon appétit!

**Nutrition:** 171 Calories; 17g Fat; 2g Total Carbs; 7g, Protein; 4g Sugars

# Mushroom Delight with Barbecue Sauce

**Prep Time:** 10 minutes | **Serve:** 4

- 1 pound brown mushrooms

Barbecue sauce:
- 10 ounces tomato paste
- 1 cup water
- Sea salt and ground black pepper, to taste 1/2 teaspoon porcini powder 1 teaspoon shallot powder
- 1 teaspoon garlic powder
- 1 teaspoon mustard seeds
- ½ teaspoon fennel seeds
- 2 tablespoons lime juice
- 1 tablespoon coconut aminos
- A few drops liquid Stevia
- 1 teaspoon liquid smoke

1.Clean and slice the mushrooms; set them aside.

2.Add the remaining ingredients to your Instant Pot andstir to combine; stir in the mushrooms.

3.Secure the lid. Choose "Manual" mode and High pressure; cook for 4 minutes. Once cooking is complete, use a natural pressure release; carefully remove the lid. Serve warm.

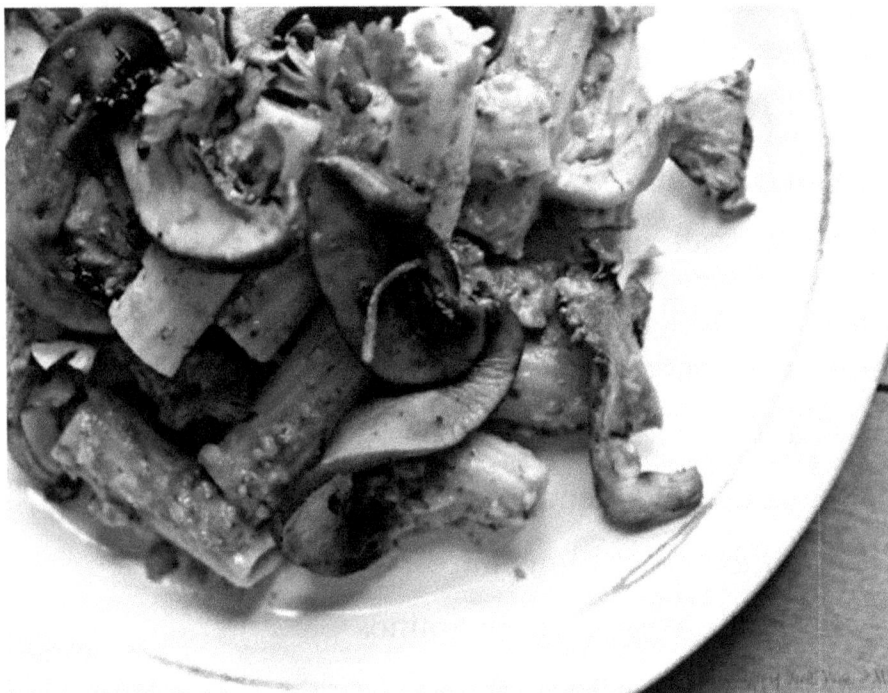

# Mediterranean Zoodles with Avocado

**Prep Time:** 10 minutes | **Serve:** 2

- 2 tablespoon olive oil
- 2 tomatoes, chopped
- 1 teaspoon garlic, smashed
- 1 tablespoon fresh rosemary, chopped 1/2 cup fresh parsley, roughly chopped 1/2 cup water
- 3 tablespoons almonds, ground
- 1 tablespoon apple cider vinegar
- 2 zucchinis, spiralized
- ½ avocado, pitted and sliced
- Salt and ground black pepper, to taste

1.Add olive oil, tomatoes, garlic, rosemary, parsley, water, ground almonds, and apple cider vinegar to your Instant Pot.

2.Secure the lid. Choose "Manual" mode and High pressure; cook for 5 minutes. Once cooking is complete, use a natural pressure release; carefully remove the lid.

3.Divide zoodles between two serving plates. Spoon the sauce over each serving. Top with avocado slices.

4.Season with salt and black pepper to taste. Bon appétit!

# Chinese Vegan Stew

**Prep Time:** 20 minutes | **Serve:** 4

- 2 tablespoons sesame oil
- 1 red onion, chopped
- 1 teaspoon ginger-garlic paste
- 1 celery stalk, sliced
- 1 carrot, sliced
- 3 cups brown mushrooms, sliced
- 2 ripe Roma tomatoes, puréed
- 1 cup vegetable broth, preferably homemade
- 1 (12-ounce) bottle amber beer
- 2 bay leaves
- ½ teaspoon caraway seeds
- ¼ teaspoon cumin seeds
- ½ teaspoon fenugreek seeds
- Sea salt and ground black pepper, to taste 1 teaspoon Hungarian hot paprika 1 tablespoon soy sauce

1.Press the "Sauté" button to heat your Instant Pot. Heat the sesame oil and cook the onions for 2 to 3 minutes or until tender and translucent.

2.Now, add ginger-garlic paste, celery, carrot and mushrooms; continue to cook for a further 2 minutes or until fragrant.

3.Add the remaining ingredients, except for soy sauce.

4.Secure the lid. Choose "Manual" mode and High pressure; cook for 10 minutes. Once cooking is complete, use a quick pressure release; carefully remove the lid.

5.Ladle into individual bowls, add a few drizzles of soy sauce and serve warm. Bon appétit!

**Nutrition:** 136 Calories; 3g Fat; 4g Total Carbs; 6g, Protein; 5g Sugars

# Chunky Autumn Chowder

**Prep Time:** 10 minutes | **Serve:** 4

- 1 ½ tablespoons olive oil
- 1 leek, chopped
- 2 cloves garlic, smashed
- 1 parsnip, chopped
- 1 celery stalk, chopped
- 4 cups water
- 2 bouillon cubes
- ½ pound green cabbage, shredded
- 1 zucchini, sliced
- 2 bay leaves
- ½ teaspoon ground cumin
- ½ teaspoon turmeric powder
- 1 teaspoon dried basil
- Kosher salt and ground black pepper, to taste 6 ounces Swiss chard

1.Press the "Sauté" button to heat your Instant Pot. Heat the olive oil and cook the leek for 2 to 3 minutes or until it is softened.

2.Add the other ingredients, except forSwiss chard, to the Instant Pot; stir to combine well.

3.Secure the lid. Choose "Manual" mode and High pressure; cook for 3 minutes. Once cooking is complete, use a quick pressure release; carefully remove the lid.

4.Add Swiss chard and cover with the lid. Allow it to sit in the residual heat until it is wilted.

5.Discard bay leaves and ladle into soup bowls.

**Nutrition:** 99 Calories; 5g Fat; 2g Total Carbs; 2g, Protein; 4g Sugars

# Chowder with Zucchini and Leek

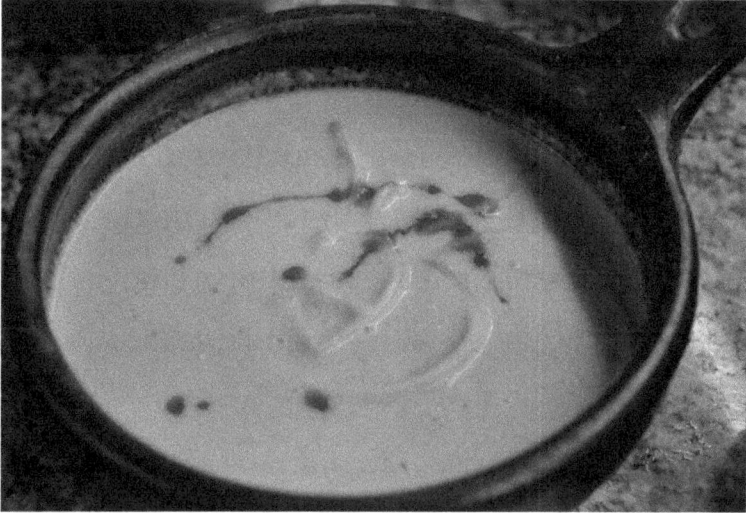

**Prep Time:** 15 minutes | **Serve:** 4

- 2 tablespoons coconut oil
- 1 medium-sized leek, thinly sliced
- 1 zucchini, chopped
- 2 garlic cloves, crushed
- Sea salt and ground black pepper, to your liking 1/2 teaspoon cayenne pepper 4 cups vegetable stock
- ¼ cup coriander leaves, chopped

1.Press the "Sauté" button to heat your Instant Pot. Heat the coconut oil and sauté the leeks, zucchini, and garlic.

2.Next, stir in the salt, black pepper, cayenne pepper, and stock.

3.Secure the lid. Choose "Manual" mode and High pressure; cook for 8 minutes. Once cooking is complete, use a natural pressure release; carefully remove the lid.

4.Serve warm garnished with coriander leaves.

**Nutrition:** 90 Calories; 4g Fat; 9g Total Carbs; 2g, Protein; 5g Sugars

# Baked Lamb Stew

**Prep Time:** 15 min | **Cook Time:** 1 h 10 min | **Serve:** 4

For Lamb Marinade:

- 3 large garlic cloves, minced
- 1 tablespoon fresh ginger, minced
- 1 lemongrass stalk, minced
- 2 tablespoons coconut aminos
- 2 tablespoons tapioca starch
- Salt and freshly ground black pepper, to taste 2-3 pound boneless lamb shoulder, trimmed and cubed into 2-inch pieces

For Stew:

- 2 tablespoons coconut oil
- 4 shallots, minced
- 2 Thai chilies, minced
- 2 tablespoons tomato paste
- 4 large tomatoes, chopped
- 4 carrots, peeled and chopped
- 1 butternut squash, peeled and cubed

- 2 stars anise
- 1 cinnamon stick
- 1 teaspoon Chinese 5-spice powder
- 2½ cups hot beef broth

1.For lamb marinade in a large glass bowl, add all ingredients and mix well.

2.Cover and refrigerate to marinate for about 2-8 hours.

3.Preheat the oven to 325 degrees F.

4.In an oven proof casserole dish, heat oil on medium-high heat.

5.Add lamb and cook for about 4-5 minutes.

6.Reduce the heat to medium.

7.Add shallots and chilies and cook for about 2-3 minutes.

8.Stir in tomato paste and tomatoes and cook for about 1-2 minutes.

9.Add remaining ingredients and stir to combine well.

10.Cover the casserole dish and immediately, transfer into oven.

11.Bake for about 1 hour or till desired doneness.

# Haddock & Potato Stew

**Prep Time:** 15 min | **Cook Time:** 13 min | **Serve:** 4

- 2 large Yukon Gold potatoes, sliced into ¼-inch size
- 1 tbsp olive oil
- 1 (2-inch) piece fresh ginger, chopped finely
- 1 (16-ounce) can whole tomatoes, crushed ½ cup water
- 1 cup clam juice
- ¼ teaspoon red pepper flakes, crushed
- Salt, to taste
- 1½ pound boneless haddock, cut into 2inch pieces 2 tablespoons fresh parsley, chopped

Arrange a steamer basket in a large pan of water and bring to a boil.

1.Place the potatoes in steamer basket and cook, covered for about 8 minutes.

2.Meanwhile in a pan, heat oil on medium heat.

3.Add ginger and sauté for about 1 minute.

4.Add tomatoes and cook, stirring continuously for about 2 minutes.

5.Add water, clam juice, red pepper flakes and bring to a boil.

6.Simmer for about 5 minutes, stirring occasionally.

7.Gently, stir in haddock pieces and simmer, covered for about 5 minutes or till desired doneness.

8.In serving bowls, divide potatoes and top with haddock mixture.

9.Garnish with parsley and serve.

# Adzuki Beans & Carrot Stew

**Prep Time:** 15 min | **Cook Time:** 1 h 18 min | **Serve:** 4

- 2 tablespoons olive oil
- 1 large yellow onion, chopped
- 5 (½-inch) fresh ginger slices
- Salt, to taste
- 3 cups water
- 1 cup dried adzuki beans, soaked for overnight, rinsed and drained
- 4 large carrots, peeled and sliced into ¾-inch pieces
- 2 tablespoons brown rice vinegar
- 3 tablespoons tamari
- ½ cup fresh parsley, minced

1.In a large pan, heat oil on medium heat.

2.Add onion, ginger and salt and sauté for about 2-3 minutes.

3.Add water and beans and bring to a boil.

4.Reduce the heat to low and simmer, covered for about 45 minutes.

5.Arrange carrot slices over beans and simmer, covered for about 20-30 minutes.

6.Stir in vinegar and tamari and remove from heat.

7.Discard te ginger slices before serving.

8.Serve hot with garnishing of parsley.

# Black-Eyed Beans Stew

**Prep Time:** 15 m | **Cook Time:** 2 h 20 m | **Serve:** 4-5

- 2 cups dried black eyed beans, soaked for overnight, rinsed and drained
- 2 medium onions, chopped and divided
- 1 (4-inch) piece fresh ginger chopped
- 4 garlic cloves, chopped
- ¼ cup olive oil
- 2 scotch bonnet peppers
- 2 (14-ounce) cans plum tomatoes
- ½-¾ cup water
- 1 vegetable bouillon cube
- Salt, to taste

1.In a large pan of boiling water, add beans and cook, covered for about 60-90 minutes or till bens become soft.

2.In a blender, add 1 onion, ginger and garlic and pulse till a puree forms.

3.In a large pan, heat oil on medium heat.

4.Add onion and sauté for about 2-5 minutes.

5.Stir in 5 tablespoons of onion puree and cook for about 5 minutes.

6.Meanwhile in blender, add bonnet peppers and tomatoes and pulse till smooth.

7.Add tomato mixture and stir to combine.

8.Reduce the heat to low and simmer, covered for about 30 minutes, stirring occasionally.

9.Stir in beans, cube and salt and simmer for about 10 minutes.

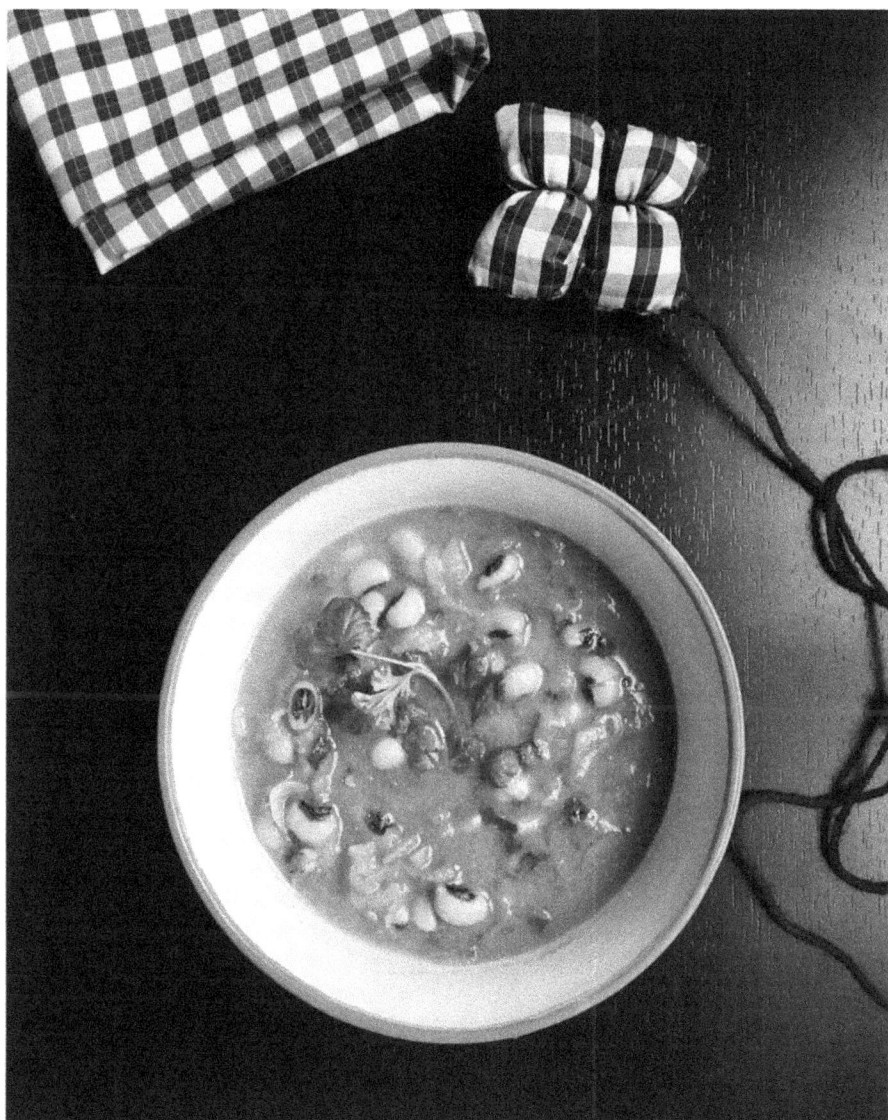